LUPUS

Advance Praise

I love WiseBetty's no-nonsense approach to healing. I can't wait to start building my "To Try" list and create my Self-care/Self-Love scale with my tribe. I'M READY!...

Mia Lyn

I wasn't sure what to expect from this book, but these remedies and tasks are so much fun and doable. With my chronic fatigue, I'm encouraged by all the support. Looking forward to day one of the movement....

Stephanie Phillips

LUPUS

Natural Remedies *for* Extraordinary Health *and* Self-Healing

WISE BETTY

NEW YORK

LONDON • NASHVILLE • MELBOURNE • VANCOUVER

LUPUS

Natural Remedies *for* Extraordinary Health *and* Self-Healing

Published in New York, New York, by Morgan James Publishing in partnership with Difference Press. Morgan James is a trademark of Morgan James, LLC. www.MorganJamesPublishing.com

ISBN 9781642793932 paperback
ISBN 9781642793949 eBook
ISBN 9781642793956 audiobook
Library of Congress Control Number: 2018914373

Cover & Interior Design by:
Christopher Kirk
www.GFSstudio.com

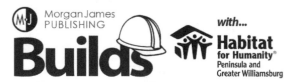

Morgan James is a proud partner of Habitat for Humanity Peninsula and Greater Williamsburg. Partners in building since 2006.

Get involved today! Visit
MorganJamesPublishing.com/giving-back

This book is lovingly dedicated
to my best friend, my twin soul, and the
love of my life, my daughter Jamishay for always
making me want to become a better version of myself.
When the world is trying to crush me down, you give
me the strength to fight back and keep aiming high.

-

To the other love of my life, my mom Miladiys.
Thank you for believing in me and being proud of
me. I've waited all my life to hear you say that.

-

To my three babies with paws, Lulu, TyTy, and
Sophie, thank you for always surrounding me with
unconditional love, kisses, and cuddles when I need
it the most. I didn't rescue you, you rescued me.

-

And lastly, my baby girl with paws Suzy,
RIP my beautiful Angel. I feel you watching over me.
Just sit tight and wait for mommy in heaven.

Table of Contents

Foreword

I've had the great pleasure of getting to know WiseBetty over the last year and learning about her incredible passion for helping others that struggle with finding real, helpful solutions for their autoimmune condition. She genuinely cares with deep heartfelt compassion as she focuses on healing one person at a time.

I'm convinced that there is no better teacher or authority than one who actually healed themselves from Lupus or another autoimmune condition on their own. Compared to so many healthcare practitioners or coaches that only learned what was taught to them, WiseBetty offers a unique perspective as a health and wellness consultant and shares her valuable secrets to natural healing while teaching us how to attune ourselves to our bodies' needs.

There really is nothing stronger than a woman that has rebuilt herself, and then takes the initiative to pave the way as a beacon of <u>light</u> for others. WiseBetty's calling to inspire others deeply resonates with me because I too suffered for many years and healed myself from various health issues, including a near-death experience, while making significant clinical research breakthroughs and discoveries in the process. Suffering can be a blessing in disguise if it means offering hope and proven solutions in order to help others reach greater levels of health and vitality.

WiseBetty makes applying her personal recommendations easy to learn, practical and fun. Now is the time to put this information into action. The people in her tribe are nurtured like her own family and have gone on to develop healthier habits. Self-care is how you take your power back, and please remember that you can't pour from an empty cup. Take good care of yourself first and dare to begin.

Many blessings on your healing journey!

Dr. John Foley
Founder of BodyCures
www.bodycures.com

Introduction

" I Got You!"

I was recently asked why I decided to write this book. It seemed like an easy question at the time, but I found myself struggling to come up with just one good solid answer, cause to be honest, I wrote this book for many reasons. I wrote this book, so I could have a record with a timeline of events that led to my Lupus diagnosis. I wrote this as a book of beginner's remedies and recipes for healing. I wrote this book, so when I'm no longer here, my daughter will have a safe place to turn when she experiences her own autoimmune flare-ups and episodes. But the one most important reason why I wrote this book is you. You're the reason I wanted to share my story. You're the reason why all these years of suffering will not be in vain. With no one to turn to for guidance when I first found out I had Lupus, I had to find ways to naturally heal myself on my own. With the increase of doctor's visits and no health insurance, I basically had to be my own guinea pig and learn methods to self-heal. It's been a tough, hard, long, and lonesome journey, one that no one should travel alone, so I want you to remember something:

- When people tell you, "Seriously, I think it's all in your head," just know…
  I BELIEVE YOU.
- When people ask, "Depression? Why can't you just be happy?" just know…
  I BELIEVE YOU.
- When people say, "You sleep way too much, you're just lazy," just know…
  I BELIEVE YOU.
- When doctors are saying, "There is nothing wrong with you," just know…
  I BELIEVE YOU.
- When doctors are saying, "It's hormonal changes and stress," just know…
  I BELIEVE YOU.
- When your doctor is misdiagnosing you for the fifteenth time, just know…
  I BELIEVE YOU.
- When people tell you, "I don't believe you, you don't look sick," just know…

I BELIEVE YOU.
- When people tell you, "You're just doing all this for attention," just know…
I BELIEVE YOU.
- When people accuse you of acting like a crazy hypochondriac, just know…
I BELIEVE YOU.
- When people accuse you of just not wanting to get any better, just know…
I BELIEVE YOU.
- When you're entertaining thoughts of suicide because of pain, just know…
I BELIEVE YOU.

When you're sitting in a dark room wondering who to turn to, just know… I GOT YOU!

I decided to write this book to you because I want to invite you to join me on an amazing, powerful and fun self-healing journey. With me, you will discover the secrets to soothing all your auto-immune symptoms. Whether you are currently experiencing an episode or just coming out of a flare up, these secrets will now be your guiding light, the force that will lead you to experience full remission of your illness. By exploring delicious and easy ways to use your food as medicine, while incorporating science-backed natural nutrients and powerful healing remedies and supplements into your new daily life-style routine, you will once again discover what it feels like to live life pain free all over again. By the end of this book, you will not only be leaving with an arsenal of healthy healing information, but you'll also be joining a strong support system of people on this journey with you.

No matter where you are in your life right now, I want you to join me. Now is the perfect time to start stepping into your better healthier self. Now is the perfect time for you to accept my invitation and come join my "ME NOW" self-healing warrior movement. Your time for a joyous pain free life started the minute you picked up this book and will continue as we walk this journey together.

Oh yes, one other thing before we begin, there's just something I must ask of you in return, in order for this self-healing warrior movement to succeed. By stepping into your better healthier self, I'll require just one very important favor of you. I'm asking that during our self-healing journey together, you stop and take the time to look at yourself not with critical eyes, but instead with honest, nurturing, caring eyes. Because self-care, self-love, determination, patience, and an open mind are going to be the powerful building blocks necessary for making your self-healing journey a success.

Here's to you healing forward with purpose…. Cheers!

PART ONE:
Change Your Mind Change Your Story

"Often the soul always knows what to do to heal itself, the challenge is how to silence the mind…"
~Caroline Myss

CHAPTER 1

Lupus: My "Me Now" Journey

I could sit here and start this book with my first diagnosis and all the meds I've tried and taken; I can talk about all the negative feedback I've experienced; and I can also talk about not being understood or believed; or about the million times I've been misdiagnosed and dismissed as an attention getting hypochondriac; and so on and so forth, but that's not where my heart wants to go with this. Yes, it's important to touch upon these moments for clarity sake and as a road-map so you can see how I got from point A to point B, however that's not how I'm going to approach this. What I will be doing instead is mostly sprinkling these moments throughout the book as it relates to the topic at hand. What I want to do with this chapter instead is have you get to know the real me and how my brain works. By getting to know me this way, you'll understand how and why I was able to find that loophole to healing myself (a loophole that can help guide you into healing yourself from this horrible epidemic as well), and I'll also discuss how I partnered with the Law of Attraction (LOA), especially during my darkest moments when I just needed someone to take the wheel for a bit.

When I look back at my years with Lupus, what I see is a dis-ease that is more of a blessing than a curse. Now, for those of you reading this who are in the midst of an excruciating episode, just stay with me because I know what you're thinking, "What in the name of autoimmune diseases is she talking about?" Well, what I realized during every mentally and physically challenging episode, every self-esteem destroying flare up, straight through every moment of debilitating sadness and suicidal thoughts, that there was always a call to action. In those moments, there was a voice, a presence with me that held my hand tightly as I dangled in that dark place, telling me, "I got you, and when you're ready, we'll climb the next mountain together." Now, because you're living with an autoimmune disease, the only call to action you're likely to experience is wanting to disappear from the world into a dark room and go straight to bed, so let me explain what I mean by a call to action.

I have always been what I like to call a "social loner." Whether it's surfing videos and binge-watching show episodes, grabbing a glass of wine and reading a good book while cuddling with my children with paws, or even blasting my music in my car and singing at the top of my lungs (I love doing this with my daughter, she gets me), I love my own company enough to want it 95 percent of the time. I don't have a problem being alone. I like not feeling like I'm responsible for everyone's good-time, or worse, their entertainment. Plus, if I'm experiencing a moment where I can feel my body shutting down and need to rest, I don't have to feel guilty about it. I know it isn't anyone's fault that I feel this way and it certainly isn't my responsibility to entertain anyone, but that's the care giver in me, who always takes me away from my "Me Now" warrior mindset. Perhaps you feel what I'm saying because you prefer spending time by yourself as well.

So how can being a social loner help you on your self-healing journey? Because it's in these moments of solitude that you can hear that inner voice telling you, you can do this; you can heal this; you can keep going. I can't begin to tell you how many times I looked forward to these moments of solitude, because what it taught me was to stop and look at my life, so I could witness these moments where I'd be putting myself last.

Putting yourself last is like putting an oxygen mask on everyone else on the airplane before you reach up and grab a mask for yourself. How can you possibly be present to heal yourself and others when you are basically taking yourself out of the healing equation with your actions? Actions that say, "I don't count." I developed the "Me Now" warrior movement as a thank you and an acknowledgment to my life's experience with the LOA. I wanted to let the universe know that I heard its message. When you're called to action in your healing, jumping on the "Me Now" train is basically YOU telling yourself, and a higher power, that yes you hear the message, yes you got the message, and that "Yes you're on it!"

Now here's the rub, I can guarantee to you that I wouldn't have been able to receive this call to action or think outside the box if I were feeling good or in remission, because in those moments of "feeling normal and good" I would've probably taken that moment for granted. But instead what I learned, through those character-building moments of excruciating pain, was to embrace my remission as my trophy moment and as my warrior badge for taking positive action in my healing. One thing is always guaranteed, out of the darkness you'll always find yourself ten steps further along into your self-healing journey. And as you embrace the "Me Now" warrior movement, you'll always know that a hand will be there to guide you on your way.

I'm excited to be that hand that reaches out to you and walks with you on your path when you're in those moments of darkness. Remember we're in this together (and by no means am I dismissing or invalidating where you are right now by not focusing on the suffering and pain you're experiencing as a victim of this epidemic), but I don't want to focus on what you already know and instead help you change your story. Whether you're in remission or experiencing a flare up and are deep in a painful episode, or if you're just not sure what's going on in your body between conflicting and confusing diagnosis, if you have any ailments that desire natures healings and remedies then it's time to embrace your "Me Now" warrior moment and focus on healing forward.

Before we begin your healing, in chapter two I'll briefly get into why I believe that most autoimmune dis-eases are like chameleons testing our resolve. Lupus, what I like to term as "The Dis-ease of a Thousand Faces," is like the Da Vinci Code of auto-immune disorders. It's constantly giving clues and hints about why, where and when to begin our healing, and at the same time being allusive with the how. This is where my years of self-experimentation and experience can help you achieve your self-healing goals.

CHAPTER 2
The Dis-ease of a Thousand Faces

"Part of the healing process is sharing with other people who care…"
~Psychic Therapist

When people hear that you have Lupus, most of the time they look at you with these blank stares and always answer with an, "Oh … so what is that anyway?" Or my favorite, a blank stare with no reaction at all, as if you just told them you had a headache. People will understand other autoimmune dis-eases. For instance, they will react when you tell them you have Lymes dis-ease (sorta), even though they have no idea how it exactly destroys your body. They understand MS, but only when it has already outwardly physically affected the patient, and they've heard of Crohn's and Graves dis-ease but the only thing they know of the disease is that they're glad they don't have it. But when it comes to Lupus, because it was considered an "ethnic/other" disease mostly affecting black and brown people, nobody was really interested in knowing anything further about it. Even doctors were indifferent about it, and still are even though Lupus affects over 1.5 million Americans, with more than 200,000 US cases per year.

Although it has now crossed over to all nationalities, ethnicities, and races, doctors still don't know where to start in healing this dis-ease and instead find ways to feed the symptoms with harsh drugs that initially help, but then become too toxic for the body's system to handle and eventually starts to fight back. The reason doctors react this way with Lupus, I believe, is because it can be a very illusive, vague, and hard dis-ease to diagnose. There are way too many false positives and false negatives associated with trying to diagnose Lupus, and with such a small percentage of actual definite diagnosis given yearly to patients, it's a clear telltale sign that we still have some ways to go for a real medical cure.

With that said, my best advice from this point forward is for you to become a strong advocate for yourself. The best thing I did for myself was to keep a record of my symptoms, episodes, and my flare-ups (if you're going to be incorporating the doctor route into your self-healing journey, I highly recommend this). It's important to be able to show your doctors a pattern of your symptoms, plus it shows that you mean business. Unless you walk in with three or more Lupus symptoms all at the same time, as it happened to me, it will take a while for you to get a proper diagnosis. It was only after I was sent to the hospital because of a full-blown staph infection from the lesions my family doctor incorrectly treated, that my doctor finally believed that the diagnosis of Lupus given to me by a holistic doctor was correct.

So, with that said, let's see why an autoimmune disease like Lupus (an inflammatory disease whose immune system attacks its own tissues), is so difficult for doctors to treat and many times diagnose. Let's break down the three most common early symptoms (and there are many but we'll start with these) affecting Lupus sufferers.

Vague Symptom #1 - Fatigue

Fatigue is at the top of the list of the three critical early symptoms of this dis-ease, but it's probably the #1 most debilitating symptom of Lupus. Unfortunately, fatigue is also one of those symptoms that fall under every other negative ailment known to man. Once your body is on the defensive and wants to protect you, it slows you down and kinda tries to get you out of the way, so it can heal you. One of the ways it does that is sometimes by putting you through the feeling of extreme debilitating exhaustion. The feeling is almost the same as being sedated by general anesthetics except you're awake and feel the pain.

The difference with Lupus fatigue and "regular" fatigue is that Lupus fatigue does not go away no matter how much rest you get because it weakens you at a deep cellular level. Unfortunately, because fatigue ranges anywhere from all sorts of diseases and viruses, to hard work or a night of heavy partying, try showing up to your doctors' appointment and telling them about your debilitating fatigue. Chances are they won't even take any blood work (unless you insist), and if you're a woman, unfortunately they'll either blame it on your lifestyle or blame it on stress and your hormones. In essence, they slam the door shut to any other medical possibility.

Vague Symptom #2 - Joint/Arthritis Pain

Joint pain, whether it be rheumatoid or osteo, is another symptom that I would keep at the top of the three critical symptoms of this disease. The reason is because the pain is so agonizing that you feel like your whole body is literally in a vice. Couple that with your fatigue and you literally feel like you're dying. It's the kind of pain that comes on from one day to the next with absolutely no warning, while progressing downhill very quickly. Depending on where in your body it begins, it can either slowly prevent you from walking or make you barely able to move your hands to the point of feeling immobile.

I unfortunately allowed the stress I was facing at the time to take over my life. I allowed stress and doubt to change my healing story, and as a result, it gave way for my Lupus to completely debilitate my body. My pain got so severe that I couldn't sit for more than five minutes at a time because then I wouldn't be able to stand up. My body would lock in place. I was also losing back support from the pain in my lower back and knees, and when I tried tightening my core to help myself stand up, it would only make the pain in my lower back worse, forcing me to stand most of the time. But then I couldn't stand for long periods of time because of the fatigue and the pain in my joints. I was a mess with joint pain.

Looking back, I remember sitting in meetings and waiting until everybody left the room before I attempted to stand because there was no way I was going to be able to get up without looking like I was 90 years old. I would have to get up by holding onto a table or the back of a nearby chair. I would bend over, then slowly raise my torso up while I felt the agonizing pain of every nerve in my body being shocked. My knees would get stiff from sitting while my feet would swell from the lymphedema that had settled from the lack of circulation in my legs. So, sitting was the enemy, standing was the enemy, and laying down was the enemy. The only thing that felt somewhat okay, once I got to warm up my muscles and joints, was walking and keeping everything in motion. That was the thing that kept me able to feel somewhat human.

If I stopped for more than ten minutes, the feeling of being in a vice would begin to stiffen my joints and muscles again. The stress would then immediately begin to shoot pain to my lower back and the cycle would start over again. When I went to my doctor all he saw was someone who walked in looking somewhat normal and in not that much pain. He would then look at me as if he were examining someone who was experiencing imaginary symptoms because of stress or dealing with someone unhappy with life. That's when I knew this doctor wasn't there to help me. And he certainly couldn't help me if I couldn't help myself. At that moment I decided to change my story, to move away from being the victim and instead become the detective and healer of my own body. That's when I decided to take my healing into my own hands.

Because joint pain is another one of those symptoms that could range anywhere from rheumatoid arthritis to even lifting too many weights at the gym, unless you come in all twisted into your doctor's office you're going to be sent home with nothing but Tylenol. At best you'll probably get one of those, "Sorry I can't do anything for you, maybe you should go see a rheumatologist," kinda deals leaving you back at square one.

Vague Symptom #3 - Butter Fly Rashes and Lesions

Several years ago, I woke up with a lesion between my breasts. It was itchy and painful, but I just thought that maybe I was reacting to a mosquito bite, as I'm allergic to mosquito bites. I started to get one of my fevers and it started to get hot around my torso. Several hours later, when I went to see what was going on with my rash, the lesions had spread to the whole entire right side of my torso, slowly climbing up my right arm. I was being eaten alive by some skin bacteria. I called the doctor for an emergency visit. When I got there, he said he'd never seen anything like it before. He said that even though he didn't think it was shingles, he was going to give me meds and a cream for shingles to see if we could at least prevent it from spreading and stop the burning. It was a shot in the dark, and even though it didn't sound right to me, I was so desperate that I agreed to everything he said. I just wanted the pain and burning and fevers to stop.

Well fast forward three days from taking the meds, the skin on my torso started to turn even redder from the burning and itchier from being eaten up alive by this bacterium. I was lethargic and had a fever. I went back to the doctor who sent me to the hospital where I saw a dermatologist who took a biopsy and found that the side effect from these meds caused my lesions to morph into a full-blown staph infection. I was immediately put on antibiotics, topically and orally, and also given Prednisone.

So once again, there I was with another one of the three top critical symptoms of Lupus, but it alone couldn't help me get a proper diagnosis.

Butterfly rashes and skin lesions are the third tell-tale signs of Lupus and the third on my list of top three critical early signs. They call it the butterfly rash because it's mostly been recognized on the upper parts of the cheeks and nose, but it can actually appear on any part of the lower half of your face. Mine appeared on the sides of my cheeks and the bottom part of my mouth when I did get skin flare-ups. They were painful; they burned and almost always messed with my self-esteem. But again, these are symptoms that can be confused with eczema, psoriasis, cystic acne, and a host of other skin conditions. The lesions however, are a different story in the sense that if you have them, they will consider a biopsy depending on how severe they look.

The issue with lesions is that, if not taken care of quickly, it can go into your blood stream (like shingles and poison ivy) and cause an infection. When you have Lupus, an infection is not something you ever want to provoke. The lesions feel something like chicken pox along with the fever, except you feel like you're being eaten alive. An improper diagnosis and treatment can lead to a painful staph infection, which is what happened to me.

Many moons ago when I was a teenager, I had gone back and forth to several physicians, and at the end of the day they never found anything wrong and always blamed it on my teenage hormones. Thankfully, in one of my newly recommended holistic doctor visits, I was fortunate enough to have several symptoms flare up all at once on my way to my appointment. This enabled me to get a confirmed diagnosis. Honestly, I never went for a second opinion after that for fear of entering another round of run-arounds and doctor's bills. I grabbed onto that diagnosis and ran with it. Even though I had no idea what he was talking about, when I asked this Chinese holistic doctor to break the dis-ease down in laymen terms for me, so I would know how to proceed, he said, "Your body is basically allergic to itself, and it will fight itself." His words were short and to the point, exactly the information I wanted and needed to begin my healing.

Now, over the years, I've learned to expand the breakdown of this dis-ease to give a better visual of its effects on the system. So, in a nutshell your body gets allergic to itself making your immune system think that you are the enemy. It feels that it must save you from yourself, therefore attacking its own defenses (aka its allies). In turn your defenses are now forced to fight against their own platoon in a never-ending effort to defend itself. Your body then falls into a slow inflammatory cycle of death that will eventually begin to destroy the function of your organs (which, by the way, were forced into this battle unwillingly, then work themselves on dangerous rounds of overtime, with no meal breaks, to their eventual demise). This is why it is critical for you to help reprogram your system, so it no longer sees you as the enemy that it must overload with its inflammatory ammunition.

Now here's where you have the chance and power to change your story. Listen, I totally get it, I get that it's important to get validation from a professional, remember I've been there. But validation, I found, isn't enough. All it does is confirm that you're not going crazy and that your symptoms are not just in your head. But then there's the long road of validating your symptoms with a name, which can take years. If wanting to know is more important than wanting to take matters into your own hands and begin your self-healing journey, then this book is definitely not for you, because accepting my invitation is confirming that you're ready to take self-healing actions now. Accepting my invitation is you saying, I'm sick and tired, of being sick and tired!"

One thing I learned over the years is that some doctors don't really want to heal patients. They can't make money from healing you; they can only make money by temporarily trying to help you resolve your immediate problems, which are your symptoms. In order to self-heal, you must start with trust: trusting yourself; trusting the journey; trusting your coach; and in turn trusting the process.

Lessons in Summary

I wanted to summarize this chapter for two reasons: As Lupus patients, we are constantly being discouraged from discovering natural organic self-healing remedies, while being told that only pharmaceuticals can successfully treat our symptoms; and we're also told that there is no possible cure for this dis-ease and to just please accept that narrative.

The lesson in this chapter that I hope to convey is of the importance of being in command of your healing but also the importance of recognizing that first it begins by changing your story. The day when I decided once and for all to change my story from victim to self-healer, was the day I was the sickest I'd ever been in my life. And when I finally made the choice to get back on my self-healing journey, (the "Me Now" Warrior Movement), that's when the universe opened up its arms and said, "Your wish is my command." Changing my story became the first step to discovering the secrets to healing. Now it's your turn and I can take you there.

CHAPTER 3

Getting Rid of Self-Limiting Beliefs and Habits

"Out of suffering have emerged the strongest souls..."
~The Healing Center

When I was sixteen, I remember riding the train with my sister. We were having a fun time laughing and making jokes, then the train stopped at one of the first busy stations on the Manhattan Broadway line. As the doors opened, I suddenly felt the walls start caving in on me. I felt hot, faint, and terrified. I couldn't breathe and if I didn't get off that train I felt I was going to lose my mind. My sister and I ran off the train as the doors closed behind us. I stood on the platform holding onto one of the columns for dear life. That was the beginning of my 16 debilitating years of having panic disorder. That was a strange year for me where I started having early symptoms of Lupus, but they appeared and disappeared so often

21

that I started to wonder if I was losing my mind. One minute my whole body would swell, and the next minute I would faint and wake in a puddle of sweat shivering and confused.

Fast forward three years later, at 19 years old, I'm sitting in the last doctor's office I promised myself I would sit in. For three years I went from doctor to doctor, and emergency rooms, and all I got was that it was just teenage angst and puberty. This day was different as I was finally deathly ill in a doctor's office, and not sitting there after an episode trying to explain my symptoms. I was living sick in the moment, in real time in front of a holistic doctor, where I was experiencing three critical symptoms all at once. YES! He then gave me my Lupus diagnosis and I was off on my happy and sick merry way. I finally felt human and not insane. From that day on, I grabbed myself by the boot straps and started my years of self-experimentation and self-healing.

During this time, I was still experiencing paralyzing bouts of panic attacks and anxiety that I couldn't shake off because I had no idea what it was. I couldn't talk to anyone about it, so I did what most people with panic disorder do and that's avoid places, people, and things that triggered me. I learned grounding methods, so I could function but spent most of my time in my apartment binge watching movies while trying to find a cure for my dis-ease.

I was stuck in that wanting-to-be-cured phase. I joined groups, seminars, and anything that could help me find myself and also feed my desire to be cured. I always felt awkward as if I were standing outside of myself looking in, but these places made me feel normal. I always felt disconnected from my body and just slightly off center mentally, but these places gave me purpose. The only thing that kept me going for years was my want and determination to know what was happening to my body and mind. I would never describe myself as sad, just cautious. I was not necessarily suicidal but always felt like I took up space. I tried mediums, therapists, and basically lived in the self-help section of Barnes and Nobles. I spent my time people watching. I people watched because I was trying to find parts of myself in them, so I could try and put the pieces together of who I was. I wanted to find myself in them through my own eyes, and not through their judgments of me.

Fast forward years later, I finally got the answers I was looking for. For years I spent my life in a state of self-limiting beliefs about myself and my health, which as a result, developed into self-limiting habits that basically had me spinning my wheels. You see I never believed that I could "cure" myself or really feel normal. For years my wanting to want gave me purpose. My search gave me a reason to get up in the morning. Being sick gave my life meaning and something to fix. Having Lupus and panic disorder was my self-identifier. I knew that girl intimately and she made me feel safe. But then reality hit, and I realized that I couldn't successfully heal if my self-identifier was my illness. I was giving power to something that I was only wishing away but mentally holding on to.

Maybe after reading my story you can see a part of yourself in me. Are there stories you've told yourself about your body, your health, your happiness, and your life that have kept you from seeking alternative forms of healing or reaching your health potential? Have you kept yourself in endless cycles of doctor's visits spinning your wheels? Or worse, have you accepted your prognosis as your identifier?

Below I want you to take a minute and reflect on the following questions:

Self-Limiting Story
- What is your self-limiting story?
- What are your self-limiting identifiers and beliefs?
- What self-limiting habits have you developed to validate your self-limiting story?
- Are you still wanting to want, or are you ready for change?
- How do you want to change your story to a more empowering narrative than what you've already subscribed too?
- Are you ready to heal forward?

If you're ready to change your story and see yourself as the driving force behind your healing, then let's get to it. Keep reading!

PART TWO:
Heal Your Body - Heal Your Mind

"I now free myself from all fears and doubts…"
~Louise Hay

CHAPTER 4
Knowing Your Nutritional Needs

O kay so enough stories. From this point forward, it's healing time. It's remedy time. Is it safe to assume that you have made the decision to climb aboard the "Me Now" Warrior train to begin your self-healing journey with me? If so, then let's talk nutrition. Although food should be your main priority when it comes to medicine and nutrition, it would be foolish of me to tell you that food alone will be enough for you to gather most of your nutritional needs to self-heal.

In this chapter I will be listing many of the science-backed nutritional supplements along with other forms of nutritional remedies for you to start creating and preparing your very own nutrition cocktails. I won't be able to list them all, so I will only be listing the supplements and remedies that I feel you should consider adding to your cocktail list to ensure that you're starting from a strong place in your healing. Building a strong supplemental foundation is key.

When Susan came to see me she was frustrated, exhausted and in excruciating pain. She was numb from the sadness and discouraged from her inability to heal herself. She'd been from doctor to doctor and every visit put her back at square one. She wanted help and answers, none of which she was getting, and the meds she was taking were ripping a hole in her stomach. She would've tried anything to make herself feel better. After listening to her we came up with a cocktail list and remedies for her to try out, and within 10 days she came to me and said how much better she felt. Her lymphedema was gone. She was able to open and close her hands without joint pain and she started to experience more energy. I shared with her supplements and remedies that I had tried and prepared for myself that had given me good results. A full list will be available for you to review and download, with full descriptions and DIY remedies on my Facebook group.

When you begin preparing your nutritional cocktails, it's always good to start by assuming your body needs everything. I have always trusted my inner voice and was always open to suggestions. If someone would tell me, "Oh my God, I have been taking such-and-such supplement, or this combination of such-and-such has me pain free," I would immediately put it on my "To Try" list. So just keep an open mind, do your research, consult your physician if you must, and remember to keep healing forward.

So here are just some of the supplemental nutrients that have done wonders for me and my clients to help reverse symptoms and flare-ups. You will notice that the main properties these nutrients have in common are that they all fall under the antioxidant category and have anti-inflammatory properties that help our bodies with oxidative stress. So, when shopping for your cocktails, just remember the acronym (AAOS), which stands for; Antioxidant, Anti-inflammatory, and Oxidative Stress. For Lupus sufferers, these are the critical properties you'll need to look for in your nutrients when you're preparing any health cocktail. These properties help us reprogram our system and help us repair cells and reduce destructive inflammation while helping our bodies heal from oxidative stress.

NOTE: It is CRITICAL that you find the best quality and organic of all these nutrients and mix them with medicinal foods that will help ignite their properties. If you buy just your average commercial brands, then you're getting nothing for your money and just binders and fillers with no nutritional value for your body. BUYER BEWARE.

Supplements, Remedies, and Descriptions

Vitamin A

Originally when I started taking Vit-A, it was for my skin. I started to experience Lupus skin rashes on my cheekbones and could not find anything topical that would ease my flare ups (I even tried to apply Benadryl to my rashes, and even though it initially soothed the burning and the redness, after a while it did nothing). After a month of taking Vit-A, not only did it start reversing my flare-ups from the sun, I noticed that my sensitivity to light was slowly becoming less and less of an issue. Usually, going out on a bright sunny day felt like someone was throwing acid in my eyes. I couldn't take the sun's glare and often walked in the shade. I started to develop this bad habit of walking with my head down and squinting to avoid the painful glare. As a result, I always looked angry and confused. After several months of taking Vit-A, I started to feel normal walking around on bright sunny days with no more pain.

Vitamin A is something I highly recommend for anyone suffering from Lupus. As a very powerful antioxidant, it is fantastic at reducing inflammation that may surround your organs and relieves inflammation of lesions and skin rashes, it promotes cell growth and tissue repair, along with helping with vision sensitivity and pain.

Astaxanthin

Astaxanthin is another potent anti-oxidant that lives to destroy free radicals in your system. Astaxanthin is said to live longer in your system than most other anti-oxidants, an added benefit to your nutritional cocktails.

Vitamin B

The best form of taking a B vitamin is in a B-complex form which pretty much has all eight of these power nutrients wrapped up into one (e.g., B-1; B-2; B-3; B-5; B-6; B-7; B-9; and B-12). These vitamins and their properties combined are essential when you experience severe episodes of fatigue and muscle weakness. When you have no choice but to get to work, go to class, care for your family, or just try to be functional during the day, incorporating a B-complex into your daily routine is critical as it promotes healing and helps in the overall function of your body.

Vitamin B is great as a preventative nutrient. Like vitamin A, it's good for eye function and promotes overall cell health and growth (very important when your body begins to attack its own cells). It helps with the function of your gut and helps with brain fog, (as it's a great supporter for the health and function of your brain).

A definite B-vitamin to add to your cocktail if you prefer not using a B-complex is the B-vitamin Choline. For years I had serious issues with my liver, when I introduced Choline to my cocktails, I saw almost an overnight improvement in my liver. Choline helps export fat out of the liver and is also an anti-inflammatory. Choline is fantastic if you have developed a fatty liver or have issues with inflammation of the organs. Choline is also fantastic at reprogramming a sluggish metabolism due to inflammation.

There's another supplement that acts like Choline on steroids called Alpha-GPC. If you're experiencing organ inflammation and mental fog due to an overload of a fatty liver, add Alpha-GPC in place of the Choline. It not only gives you the same benefits as Choline, but it's also fantastic at improving mental fog and mental clarity as it supports cell membranes in the brain.

Bromelain

I couldn't NOT add a small piece on Bromelain as it is the best natural enzyme that mimics a potent pain-killer as well as a GI soother that helps break down hard to digest proteins. Bromelain is an anti-inflammatory and pain killer all in one, without the damage and side effects of a drug.

Brown Algae

Ecklonia Cava is brown algae that also helps with fatty liver and inflammation. This anti-oxidant is fast acting, so it's great when you start to suspect symptoms of fatty liver resurfacing.

Vitamin C

During my teens, because of my Lupus, every year I would get a terrible cold or flu, which always led to bronchitis. I could literally set my clock to this virus every year. After I started taking my health seriously, I found that all those years of hearing people say take vitamin C was not a joke. Vitamin C really worked for me. The trick with any supplement is making sure that you're getting good quality supplements and not just fillers. When I started to mix foods high in vitamin C, along with good quality C supplements, I eliminated colds, flus, and bronchitis out of my life for good. My body no longer gets colds or flus.

Vitamin C is probably one of the most studied vitamins of all time. Vitamin C is the most powerful antioxidant in our blood stream. It's because of its ability to protect the lungs from virus and oxidative stress that makes it the most studied vitamin of all time. Like vitamin A and the B's, vitamin C also has anti-inflammatory properties and also improves blood circulation. Taking your Vit-C when you know you're going to be seated for long periods of time, will ease the harmful effects of the oxidative stress and clotting caused by sitting. You will also notice that you will experience less stiffing of the joints as well.

Instead of buying vitamin water, I always take a C vitamin and dissolve it either in filtered water, mineral water, or seltzer water. It's fantastic if you also have issues with low blood sugar.

Chromium picolinate

With the unpredictable effects of Lupus, and heart inflammation being one of the symptoms, Chromium is a great mineral to help with levels of the fatty substance in the blood called triglycerides. Triglycerides inhibit inflammatory fatty compounds in the blood stream that tend to accumulate in the heart. To add a double punch, combine the benefits of Chromium and vitamin C, as vitamin C increases the absorption of Chromium. Note that it's best not to take with any Calcium or Iron supplement as these will prevent absorption of this mineral.

CoQ10

CoQ10 is an awesome coenzyme that helps with the fogginess and fatigue associated with Lupus flare ups. CoQ10 helps with the destructive effects of oxidative stress and also helps calm the blues associated with hormone changes. When you find yourself going in that dark hole, immediately start CoQ10. A great compliment to CoQ10 is 5-HTP a serotonin booster that calms anxiety and changes the feeling of fatigue to soothing calm and also acts as a sleep enhancer.

Vitamin D

I can't even begin to explain the dangers of being vitamin D deficient. This critical nutrient pretty much helps facilitate normal function of the immune system, especially in people with Lupus. It helps with the neurotransmitters in the brain to help with anxiety and depression (this is why people go through sadness when they are not exposed to sunny days. Fifteen minutes in the sun can give you the daily vitamin D required for healthy bones and a healthy outlook). During my Lupus episodes of joint and bone pain, I was amazed at how quickly this supplement worked at combating my bone pain, making the inflammation in my joints tolerable as it slowly helped reduce the swelling and pain as well.

Vitamin D is one of the nutrients beneficial not only for sleep but all around mental health by reducing depression. It also helps with the function of our body's ability to repair and build strong bones. As Lupus can be detrimental to both joints and bones, vitamin D is a very simple remedy that we can eventually, and rather quickly, stop taking as it teaches the body how to make its own vitamin D. This nutrient is a win-win for Lupus sufferers.

Vitamin K

For those of us susceptible to bone loss due to our illness, vitamin K is fantastic at building bones and preventing bone loss and fractures. It's also good for regulating blood issues like clotting. I used a Vitamin K cream when I was pregnant and started to develop a very painful varicose vain in my inner thigh.

A nurse recommended it to me and I applied it religiously, while also applying cold compresses to the area. After a few weeks, the varicose vain and pain was gone. What I also did was eat a lot of foods that were high in vitamin A to help in absorption of the K supplement. Foods like dark leafy greens and green tea. Foods also rich in calcium and diuretics like broccoli, red cabbage, celery, cucumber, and cauliflower help with bone health and flushing out toxins.

CalMag

CalMag is a combination of calcium and magnesium, two nutrients that go hand in hand. I remember years ago when I started doing my CalMag detoxes. Not only did it reverse my Lupus hair (which I will get into at length, no pun intended, in another chapter), but it also eliminated the tight feeling in my body that made me feel like I was in a vice. The detox helped eliminate years of pharmaceutical drugs out of my system (another topic I will get into detail about in another chapter), honestly, I could not believe the smell that was coming out of me.

Milk Thistle

Milk thistle is said to be a powerful detoxifier for your liver that acts as a natural filter purging toxins, pollutants, and heavy metals. The flavonoid, silymarin, is said to act as the filter in Milk thistle.

I used to abuse acetaminophens because I was always in pain. I guess I wanted to believe that they were harmless because they were over the counter and that they were relieving something, when in reality all they did was damage my liver. I started to develop a yellowish jaundice color to my skin and eyes because of the damage acetaminophen did. Milk thistle was a dream come true as it repaired the cells in my liver. Now taking 150-mg alone is fine but I found that supplements that help enhance glutathione have a lot of other helpful enzymes and minerals including Milk thistle. So, aim for power supplements that are all inclusive with the magic of AAOS.

Glutathione as I mentioned above, is a molecule that repairs aging tissues and prevents your immune system and toxins from harming your body. Whey protein, which you can make at home by preparing homemade yogurts, carries three helpful amino acids (cysteine, glycine, and glutamine) these amino acids stimulate liver cells and eliminate oxidative stress. If you want to stimulate the glutathione in your system take 150-mg of milk thistle.

Cellgevity

Another powerful supplement called cellgevity, with its high levels of quality Riboceine and milk thistle, also helps promote the natural production of glutathione by providing cellular support so the body can be at its optimum when detoxing and eliminating toxins. For those of you who wish to add another powerful supplement to your healing cocktail, this is one of the main supplements that you should put at the top of your list. With its science backed combination of ingredients and properties, you are guaranteed to eliminate organ and cell damaging inflammation. Cellgevity is the one nutrient that has all the ingredients and supplements I highly recommend in one supplement.

Cellgevity Healing Cocktail Properties
- RiboCeine™; Alpha Lipoic Acid; Broccoli Seed Extract; Turmeric Root Extract
- Resveratrol; Grape Seed Extract; Quercetin; Milk Thistle; Vitamin C
- Selenomethionine; Cordyceps; Black Pepper; Aloe Extract

Prenatal Multivitamin
You may wonder why I have written here prenatal vitamins. Well I learned that you don't have to be pregnant to enjoy the benefits of a prenatal nutrient. These nutrients are set up to have the right amount of healing properties not only for the mother but also for a growing fetus. I learned to have these around when-

ever I started running low on some of my other nutrients. This is my, I'm feeling lazy and don't feel like swallowing more than one pill, go to pill. Sometimes, when my body plateaus, I take my prenatal once a day, after a week or so, I return to whatever cocktail I've prescribed for myself and the effects are amazing.

Lupus is a very tricky dis-ease as it always keeps you on your toes. It has taught me to have an open mind in terms of healing and finding remedies. My body cycle, I've noticed goes around every 6 months, that means that every 6 months when things stop working, it's time to move on to the next healing remedy. It may seem like a lot of work, but it's only work if you see it as work. It's important to shift your thinking and see it as an opportunity to find other ways to nurture yourself with self-care/self-love and learn new things about your temple body. One thing's for sure and inevitable, our bodies are forever changing hormonally because we're maturing in age and mind, so why not stay ahead of the game. It would be irresponsible of us to keep our bodies stuck in old remedies, nutrients, even meds that don't align with our new body temple.

CHAPTER 5
Powerful Organ Cleanses

"I know that to help heal others,
I must first heal myself…"
~Carly Marie

L upus is the one disease that if given an opportunity to release its wrath on you, it could potentially begin to shut your body down one organ at a time. The main cause of death in Lupus patients is death by organ failure. There is a toxic line that once crossed, it cannot be reversed, so that's where proper and continuous cleansing of your liver, kidneys, gallbladder, skin, and most importantly your gut, plays a huge lifesaving role in your self-healing journey.

To combat such a tragedy to your body system, I will be listing several of my favorite organ cleansings and flushes that can help ease constipation and diarrhea, and also help promote an all-around feeling of good health, mental clarity, and emotional strength. After doing a cleanse my clients find that they are in a better frame of mind to focus on their strategies for self-healing, because the physical pain that makes them feel like their body is in a vice has subsided; they can breathe better because the cleanse has taken the edge off their depression and anxiety; and their skin and gut health gets stronger every day.

The one thing about any autoimmune dis-ease is the importance of learning that your organs function differently than everybody else's. That's why keeping your organs toxin free is how you can sense an episode coming while learning what to do to beat it to the punch and avoid a relapse. Cleansings also help your body gently eliminate waste and toxins through your skin, so your immune system can take a much-needed break from all the confusion.

Transitory Symptoms

I think it's important for me to cover what transitory symptoms are before you begin a cleanse, so you don't feel like it's either not working because you feel worse, or that you think you're dying. The first thing I do with my clients before any cleanse is have them take a stool softener or a natural tea laxative to clean out their intestines. Many people prefer to let the cleanse do this on its own, but I find it very taxing on the body when you have waste in your intestines at the start of the cleanse. I also find that you can taste the toxins in your mouth more as they're being eliminated, a taste many can't bear, which usually gives them nausea and dry heaves. When I begin a cleanse with empty bowels, I find that it gives my body an opportunity to absorb the liver cleansing supplements better, even though I may experience the symptoms of discharge or flush more intensely. I also find that it shortens the cleansing process more by having my body expel toxins faster.

Discharge, or organ flush, is basically a condition where the body experiences not only the physical elimination of toxins but also mental and emotional elimination of toxins. Symptoms become less and less the more you stick with daily natural liver cleansing foods, but when organs flush after a long time of abuse and relapses, you kinda feel overly stimulated by the effects of the pharmaceutical drugs flushing through and can taste the toxins in your mouth as if you're being poisoned.

However, symptoms may range anywhere from general fatigue; aches and pains in unusual parts of the body; fevers and chills that mimic flu like symptoms; lung discharge like mucousy fluid and post-nasal drip; unusual body odors and skin discharges (remember our skin is the largest organ in our body, eliminating old medications and even toxic thoughts in a cleanse usually comes out through the skin, creating awful skin odors and perspirations).

Another way for us to eliminate toxins faster is through our urine, which can smell worse than when we eat asparagus. Then there's the feeling of melancholy and irritability that can often be a symptom associated with a liver cleanse; and, you may experience a horrible metallic taste in your mouth that leads to bad breath no matter how much you brush. Now the good news is that, these transitory experiences only last for the first two to three days during the beginning of the cleanse (depending on how much processed food you consume).

After two days, the more toxins you release in terms of old meds and processed food from your bloodstream, the more you're going to start to feel a strong sense of clarity and almost a sense of floating, (sometimes to the point of feeling like you're tripping on acid). This is because of the old meds coming through and being filtered through your liver, and then discharging through your skin (Not everyone experiences this high, but if you do, it's important for you to find a way to ground yourself and NOT make any important decisions). This is where the love and support of others on the "Me Now" Warrior Movement come in handy.

Reaching out to other members on the healing journey "MeNow" Facebook group will put you in contact with friends who will also be experiencing the same symptoms as you, while there will be others that have already gone through the process and can help you with more tips to ground yourself. You will never heal alone. That's the beauty of this tribe. Self-care and self-love will only ever be a click away.

So here are my top favorite detox tonics to help turbo charge you into healing forward on your journey.

Liver, Kidney, Gallbladder, Gut Cleanse, and Flush

Cleanse #1~ Bone Broth Detox

My most powerful and potent organ cleanse is a 7-day bone broth cleanse. Bone broth as you know is filled with the marrow of the bone, plus its high in collagen, which is healing for the skin. Luckily, there are several ways to ingest bone broth, but my two go-to forms of ingestion are either as a smoothie or a broth with slivers of seaweed strips (seaweed has a lot of nutrients and is a great companion to any cleansing broth as it encourages elimination of stuck mucoid in your system and heavy metals).

Along with the bone broth, it's important to take a liver cleansing supplement to help get the party started. No matter which brand you use, it's important that the top main ingredients are milk thistle, turmeric, and black pepper. If there is no black pepper in your supplement, then either crush the supplement into your smoothie and add fresh crushed peppercorns or add freshly ground peppercorns in your broth as you swallow the supplement. Why fresh organic peppercorns you ask? Because peppercorns ignite the healing properties of the turmeric, which is an anti-inflammatory and anti-fungal antioxidant that works as a tool for eliminating inflammation in the kidneys, liver, and gut, while helping the gallbladder release enough bile to help flush out the toxins quicker.

When Kiah started her bone broth cleanse, she was already on day 11 of being on her new anti-depressant meds. Lupus depression and anxiety is not something that many doctors discuss because they're not in the business of depression and can't really understand how Lupus and depression/anxiety relate to one another. This leaves many Lupus sufferers in a very dark place for a very long time. Kiah's meds were giving her terrible headaches and diarrhea as her body was having a hard time adjusting to the new strength and the initial side effects. During the cleanse, so many emotional and physical toxins were being expelled from her body that she couldn't go back to her original low dose because they became ineffective. After the cleanse, she felt calmer with a new sense of mental clarity (before the cleanse, Kiah had issues with mental fogginess that made her day to day responsibilities almost impossible to handle and an overall feeling of melancholy that haunted her with suicidal thoughts). A week after her cleanse, she also began to feel an overall sense of wellbeing, something she had not experienced in a while. Could you imagine what your life would look like if you were able, as a Lupus sufferer, to experience an overall sense of emotional and mental wellbeing? This would be HUGE for Lupus sufferers.

Cleanse #2 ~ Beetroot Detox

The next remedy is not only an amazing organ cleanser, but also an awesome tasting blood purifier as well. The healing properties of beetroot are endless but, in this instance, we are using it as a cleanse to support liver function, so the liver can absorb and release nutrients to all the other necessary organs. Basically, I juice the beets, roots and all; I juice one piece of turmeric root along with fresh course grated peppercorn and a dash of cayenne pepper, then add a teaspoon of fresh lemon juice. The turmeric and other ingredients play as the anti-inflammation brigade and stimulate blood flow. This treatment along with your liver cleansing supplement can achieve an extraordinary cleansing if you follow the remedy to the letter. You must sip 8-12 ounces every two hours for three days straight. Always cleanse the colon prior to starting this remedy for optimum results. Your eyes and skin will have an amazing glow. It's worth every ounce of time spent flushing and discharging.

Note: If you don't have a juicer, that's fine, just grate the beets, add some MCT oil or Coconut oil; along with some grated turmeric and a sprinkle of fresh coarse peppercorns. Eat a little of this vitamin salad every two hours as if it was a prescription drug, along with either a clean cup of green tea, home-made Kombucha, or an apple cider vinegar spritzer. Add a fresh squeeze of lemon and you will be amazed at the effects this has on the overall health of your bodily functions and skin.

Cleanse #3 ~ Lemon Juice Fast

This is one of my go-to cleanses if I have a day of fasting after eating clean. This cleanse is pointless if all you're eating is processed foods, (which by the way is detrimental to anyone's health with Lupus). If you have to go dirty, then eat clean five days out of the week; eat anything you want at nauseum one day out of the week, (preferably on day one). Then end on the seventh day with a one-day lemon fast. It'll be refreshing, and you'll feel relaxed and alert.

Cleanse #4 ~ Avocado Fast

This is a tasty detoxifying liver cleanse that helps improve the overall health of your liver while helping the liver break down fats. You can start this five-day Avocado fast eating two avocadoes a day, (don't forget to sprinkle turmeric, pepper, and a dash of lemon juice). During this fast it's important to drink lots of water to help the liver along with flushing out the fats. Remember that all these remedies are being complimented with your liver cleansing supplements. After you feel your body using its fat storage as fuel, you can then add the above beetroot vitamin salad for two days while getting your liver acclimated to eating regular meals again. After this cleanse, I recommend eating one avocado a week for four weeks to ensure the reversal of any unknown liver damage, after the five to seven days on this fast you'll be proud of yourself for eating clean, but nothing is going to prepare you for the feeling of inner peace, calm, and an over-all feeling of being renewed.

Cleanse #5 ~ Turmeric Golden Milk

Turmeric, as I have mentioned earlier, is a powerful antioxidant with anti-inflammatory properties, (turmeric is also a blood thinner so please ask your doctor before attempting this cleanse). This is a very tasty remedy for an overall organ cleanse, but a very challenging cleanse as it is quite spicy. This cleanse is like turbo fuel, but the benefits and results are amazing. If you're one of those personalities that likes to jump in head first and throw caution to the wind like me, then this cleanse is for you. With a combination of turmeric, ginger, cayenne pepper, black pepper, cinnamon, bone broth, MCT oil or coconut oil, and raw honey, it's like you're literally taking the detox express train cleanse.

Another ingredient that I did not mention in the list above is an important ingredient that I want to discuss a little with you. So, to prepare the "milk" portion of this cleanse, we need to begin with non-dairy milks that are unsweetened. The three non-dairy milks you can combine all ingredients with are; almond milk, coconut milk, and rice milk. I do not recommend soy as a cleanse, but you may certainly use soy if you're just going to prepare the golden milk as a morning treat, but not as a detox cleanse.

For those of you who are experiencing a full blown painful Lupus episode, I would recommend for the first two days of the cleanse using filtered water, instead of any of the above-named milks, to give your body a stronger boost in eliminating inflammation around your organs and especially allowing your gallbladder to produce clean bile before introducing any non-dairy milk.

Filtered water is also good, and also recommended, if you're experiencing Lupus fevers before a cleanse. After two days, when you start to poop out what looks like chunks of gallstones, then you can switch to any of the non-dairy milks mentioned above. Here is how you're going to prepare your detox golden milk. By the way, for beginners, I recommend a full five days on this cleanse, and for those who love a challenge like me, I recommend a full seven days with one day of a vitamin salad to help re-introduce food back into your system.

Preparation
- 2 cups non-dairy milk/filtered water
- 1 tbsp turmeric

- 1 tsp ginger (powder or fresh juice)
- A pinch of cayenne pepper and black pepper
- 1 tsp of cinnamon
- ½ tsp bone broth powder
- ½ tsp MCT oil or coconut oil
- 1 tsp honey

In a sauce pan bring to a low simmer, then turn off stove. With a whisk, begin to add most of your dry ingredients. Slowly add one at a time and whisk until fully incorporated into the milk/water before adding the next dry ingredient. Now transfer the mixture into a blender and allow mixture to cool (mixture must cool before adding the honey. Heat destroys the healing properties of honey). Once cooled proceed to add the broth, MCT oil, and honey. Then blend into a nice frothy golden milk.

Drink IMMEDIATELY. You may prepare a batch in a thermos and shake vigorously before drinking if you need to be on the road or work. It won't be the same as drinking fresh out the blender but close enough. Have water handy between drinks to help your gallbladder flush out.

Note: Black pepper is a must since it activates the properties in the turmeric. Without this ingredient, you will be missing out on the benefits of this cleanse. (MCT oil will flush you out faster than coconut oil, so proceed with caution if you're not going to have a bathroom handy at all times).

A video is available to watch if you're more of a visual learner, or just want to cook a batch along with me. I also have videos showing you how to make your own almond, coconut, and rice milk for a more cost-effective way to enjoy this turbo cleanse.

Cleanse #6 ~ Apple Cider Vinegar and flavored shrub cleanse

This is another one of those organ detox cleanses that will test your taste buds. This is pretty much a straight forward cleanse that I consider a high-speed detox tonic. I recommend this turbo cleanse to my clients when they have special stressful occasions where they need to feel at their optimum health and free of joint pain. This is usually a social gathering that they'd rather not attend. Being at your self-healing optimum best is a fantastic head start to an otherwise socially anxious situation.

So, the way to start this is once in the morning and evening you will put an ounce of apple cider vinegar in a shot glass and bang it down (it WILL NOT taste good). After that, in a large water bottle, add an ounce of apple cider vinegar along with a half-ounce of lemon juice. You will be drinking four to six ounces of this turbo-tonic every two hours throughout the day for five days straight.

Shrub on the other hand is a 17th century fermented tonic that was used for medicinal purposes, but often used as a refreshing cleansing "soda" for its time. I have a video that shows you how to prepare different flavored fermented shrubs to add to your ACV cleanse for added flavor. Honestly, when you taste how good the shrub is, you will reconsider drinking regular soda (which is toxic for your immune system), and switch to this 17th century soda. Just add some club/seltzer or mineral water, and you'll have a great tasting homemade soda spritzer for pennies on the dollar.

Cleanse #7 ~ Kombucha and Shun Elixir Flush

Kombucha (a.k.a. mushroom tea), is a fermented tea filled with a colony of friendly bacteria that has been around since ancient times. Originated in Asia, it is known for its rich probiotic and anti-inflammatory properties. It is a healthy combination of friendly bacteria that once added to black or white tea, morphs into a strong medicinal vinegar elixir that helps flush out all sorts of parasites and unfriendly bacteria. Not only do you get the benefits of an army of friendly bacteria, but you also get the anti-inflammatory benefits and healing properties of the black or white tea.

Note: Using green tea is called Shun, another elixir in the family of fermented teas, but you also get the amazing properties of the green tea. Green tea is said to have one of the most powerful antioxidant properties for our bodies making it one of the healthiest tea elixirs on the planet.

Kombucha and Shun have been known to carry critical heart healthy properties for those Lupus patients who are experiencing inflammation around the heart. I don't recommend buying the store bought kombucha or shun as they may have other additives and flavorings for commercial sales. I have uploaded a DIY video for you to learn how to prepare your own Shun and Kombucha Elixir from scratch.

Many years ago, when kombucha wasn't even on the radar in America, I was making my own fermented teas. Now as you make your kombucha and Shun, you will see that your Scoby, (a Scoby is the live bacteria that feeds off the sugars to ferment the tea. It looks like a mushroom, that's why Kombucha used to be called mushroom tea) will give birth every morning.

In ancient times, the loving gesture was to gift away your new Scoby to a friend, neighbor, or stranger for medicinal purposes, or as a gesture of good health. So, my loving gesture to you is to pass on this amazing nurturing cleanse to guide you on your road to self-healing and recovery. After my clients begin a kombucha cleanse they immediately feel the benefits in their gut health. Because kombucha is so beneficial for aiding in eliminating toxins, my clients start to see a glow in their skin and a brightness in their eyes. Adding optimal organ cleanses to your monthly body cleansing regime is not only beneficial but also essential for your self-healing success.

CHAPTER 6
Life-Style Changes that can Save Your Life

"I am called to make positive changes in my life. I am deserving of love, happiness, and health. I am worthy of all things wonderful. I am not afraid of making changes in my life. Because I know these changes are for my highest good. I am gentle on myself in this time of transition. I have a clear vision of the direction that I would like my life to go in. Amidst all of this change, my heart is centered and my mind is peaceful. I take it one day at a time. I am conscious of my thought patterns..."
~Carly Marie

This chapter is probably going to be one of the shortest and quickest reads with the most lifesaving hacks in this whole book. As someone with a challenging and unpredictable autoimmune dis-ease like Lupus, one thing that

I found to be beneficial is to have a set of healthy routines that support me in keeping a positive frame of mind. Over the years, I have developed several life-saving (mental and physical), life-style changes that have helped me and my clients reverse stressful and negative moments so to avoid relapses and/or painful episodes.

Life-Style Health Hack #1

For years now, I have set my alarm 15-30 minutes prior to the actual time I should wake up. As I am awakened by my alarm, I immediately start to gently wake my mind and body by doing what I call a sound and body meditation. I begin by connecting with the sounds around me while focusing my attention on my feet, working my way up my legs, torso, arms, shoulders, neck, and face. While focusing on my body, I begin to gently move those parts of my body in an effort to loosen my muscles and bring circulation to those areas. If I feel any pain anywhere, I focus my attention on the area and begin to send healing energy to those joints and muscles.

I developed this habit from my days of being in such excruciating pain when I woke up in the mornings, that I could barely even walk to the bathroom and loosen my muscles in the shower. I found that being jolted out of bed immediately after my alarm went off, or before I had time to awaken my brain, caused a lot of mental and physical stress to my body that would result in stiffness, weakness, and an over-all feeling of discomfort. Being mindful of my body and the sounds around me gave my brain time to adjust to waking, while my gentle morning movements helped release good feeling hormones throughout my body that set my morning on a positive, relaxed vibration.

Life-Style Health Hack #2

Yes, I will agree that taking a shower the night prior to having a full day saves a lot of time and allows you to sleep in a little while longer, however there are a lot of mental and physical health benefits of showering in the morning that you may be missing out on. First of all, a morning shower is not just a rushed mindless ritual to be taken for granted, but also a Zen moment that starts your day off in a healing mode. Water has powerful healing properties that stimulate your lunges, blood circulation, and lymphatic system while wakening the oxygen in your brain. Standing under running water helps release negative energy and is a powerful mood enhancer.

My clients have literally changed the mood of their day by starting with their "Me Now" Warrior mini-spa treatment. The treatments start ten minutes before you're ready to get out of the shower, you begin with a quick hydrotherapy run. First you stretch and lift your arms above your head and cross them behind your head as if resting on a pillow. Then you open and expand your chest for a full shoulder and neck stretch. You then make the water extra hot (the hottest you can tolerate) then step into the flow allowing it to hit your armpits for one full minute, then after one full minute, immediately switch the water to ice cold, letting it hit your armpits for another minute. You must do this for five minutes per each armpit. This stimulates your lymphatic system and forces fresh oxygen into your lungs, as the extreme temperatures force you to take deep breaths in and out.

After you're done, sit wrapped in a towel on the edge of your tub or chair, close your eyes and then gently begin to slow down your breathing by inhaling through your nose and exhaling through your mouth. You're going to begin to feel tingling in your whole body from head to toe as you have just given your blood fresh morning oxygen that will help you get on with your day with a clear and alert mindful mindset. This has become the secret weapon for many of my successful client's self-care/self-love routine.

Life-Style Health Hack #3

If you ever saw the film "The Secret" one thing you should have taken away from it is the importance of gratitude and thankfulness. During my morning drive to work, I make sure to say thank you for all the nature and things surrounding me, because it's important to understand and connect to the natural healing energy that all things possess. As I drive I take it all in, showing gratitude and saying thank you on every turn. This is a small thing with amazing results. It creates a protective bubble that helps bounce off the negative energy we encounter daily. We all have moments of being sponges of negative attacks, that's just part of life. However, there are remedies as simple as gratitude and raising your vibration with sincerity in your thankfulness that can ease and lessen the effects and sometimes even keep negative moments at bay.

Isn't it awesome to know that a simple thing like gratitude and thankfulness can raise your vibrations high enough to heal you and help you rise above the stench of negativity? Raising your vibrations is another element needed to aid you in reprogramming this dis-ease. Raising your vibrations rewires the cell towers of communication in your body so, with Lupus, you no longer become the targeted enemy because your body's signals are being received at an optimum level of communication, giving your immune system the opportunity to attack the real enemies entering your body system.

Life-Style Health Hack #4

Vibrations are powerful things. When we come home from work, we have vibrations crawling all over us from the day, good or bad. Our life battery, just like our phone battery, needs to be recharged. All the conversations we have, all the encounters we face, all the errands and obstacles we experience carry with them different frequencies and vibrations that we need to release and leave outside our door. As soon as you come home from being in the outside world, you should immediately remove your outside clothing and change into cozy indoor clothes. They could be anything from a different outfit, to sweats or even your favorite pajamas. It's all to change your vibration, similar to leaving your ego and all your personal stuff at the door when you go to work, except this is the reverse. Leave the worldly stuff at the door as you enter your healing temple.

Before you switch into your comfy clothes, start with the ritual of washing your hands and face, shake off any and all negative vibrations. Water is essential because it carries a healing vibration. If you had a really bad day, and feel your Lupus symptoms being triggered, that's when you will go all out and shower all the negative thoughts and vibrations away. This is a great way to be an advocate for your health as Lupus is a great reactor to negativity that many times can send us into an episodic tailspin.

For many of my clients who have hit that dark pit of pain, they understand the importance of recharging their inner battery. Lupus bodies don't react the same as "normal" folks; we just can't fluff experiences away. We can't just run to the bar and have a few drinks to debrief. Our bodies will turn on us thinking we're the enemy, and no one suffers more than us. So, treat yourself with the same care and kindness you would treat a stranger or the one you love. It's honorable to take care of YOU first. It's powerful to say it's "Me Now" so I can take care of you with the most loving and healthiest me.

Life-Style Health Hack #5

This is the most fun health hack I'll be sharing. Every night, an hour before I go to bed, I cuddle with my babies with paws and I spend time just focusing on each one as I kiss and caress them. What I get in return is being showered with the most healing vibration of unconditional love, hugs, and kisses imaginable. Then I sit and talk with my daughter about her day or her dreams and visions of her future and we begin to imagine and visualize the outcome. We laugh and share funny memes and videos before I go and give myself my own "Me Now" treat. This could be anything from sitting on my deck with a glass of wine feeling the outdoor breeze, mentally going through all the things I am grateful for that day, to playing soft music while making a batch of homemade yogurts. The point is that I want to end my day the way I begin it, in a state of gratitude and peace. The outside world has no business in my home and in my head once I'm in my safe place where I hang my hat.

I want you to find your PLACE. Your PLACE is where you can go and find your peace. It could be one room in your house, or one corner of a room. Before you go to bed, put yourself in a frame of mind of innocence, peacefulness, mindfulness, and thankfulness. Dis-ease can't grow from a place of peace.

PART THREE:
Lupus Beauty Secrets

"Healing takes courage, and we all have courage, even if we have to dig a little to find it…"
~Healing Center

CHAPTER 7
Powerful Healing Beauty Treatments

In this chapter we are going to focus on healing beauty treatments for your skin and organs. As you know, Lupus can affect the quality of your skin with the many unpredictable rashes, lesions, and skin discolorations. I can't begin to count how many times I walked around looking jaundice with a dull tone to my skin especially during an episode. One thing I learned is if your skin looks good on the outside, they'll never know you're suffering on the inside. I am very obsessive about my skin because I know how much time and energy I need to dedicate to it once I experience a skin flare up.

I remembered when I was covered in lesions all over my torso and right arm (which by the way IS NOT contagious for those of you wondering). I was told that I would be scarred for life. Many of the topical ointments clear rashes but do nothing to heal the skin from within, so you're left with potential permanent dark scarring. I made it my mission to not let that happen to me or my clients. Till this day you would never know that I experienced those lesions unless I actually showed you the biopsy scars.

Life-Style Healing Secret #1

Let's get into beauty treatment #1, your state of mind. Yes, there will be days when your hormones are out of whack and your skin may feel a little dryer or oilier than usual, but don't fret, it's part of this disease and we can either complain about it or work with it. I choose to work with it because Lupus is happening to us every second of the day, but our healing is not only external but also internal if we choose the right mindset. Our mindful positive outlook can't be taken from us unless we allow it. Like it or not, negative vibrations make people look run down and bitter no matter how healthy they are. A negative outlook attracts negative, or negatively perceived, circumstances. Negativity is a smelly perfume to wear, and an intoxicating cancer-causing drug of choice. You're already at risk with Lupus, so bless and release negativity, and learn to reprogram your mental station to a brighter life-giving frequency.

Positivity does not have an expiration date. Clarity, mindfulness, and peace of mind is a state of being that your outer appearance will reflect to the outside world as a reflection of what you're thinking inside. Remember that thoughts become things. Understanding that thoughts have a formula that can work two ways is critical in learning how to manage your state of mind. Thoughts can either be negatively accelerated by mental and emotional abuse, neglect, surrounding yourself with negative people, and a negative life style. Or, thoughts can be nurtured and delicately preserved like a fine wine to help us rise to a higher level of awareness. It's all up to you. Allow your skin to exude your inner positivity.

Life-Style Healing Secret #2

Beauty treatment #2, the food you eat. If it's healthy to eat, then it's healthy to apply to your skin. We are taught to spend a ridiculous amount of money on creams and products, when we have a treasure trove of beauty treatments sitting in our own cabinets, counter tops, and in our refrigerators at home. The flavor of the moment right now in terms of skin health is collagen. Beauty companies charge us an exorbitant amount of money for products laced with collagen, and if you read the label, it carries with it an unusually minimal amount of the product we're being charged hundreds of dollars for. If you want collagen, then I say go directly to the source. The bones you buy at the market for bone broth soup carry a lot of collagen in the marrow of the bone, which is an amazing food source for Lupus skin.

I had a client who not only used my bone broth cleanse but also used my bone broth skin mask and in two days she noticed her skin started looking like baby skin. The little bit of redness that stayed behind looked like she had just been sun kissed versus her just getting over a debilitating self-esteem butterfly rash. Her co-workers were stunned by her transformation.

Food Sample Treatment #1

What I generally do is scrape an eighth of a teaspoon of the bone marrow, sprinkle some turmeric with a dash of pepper, and work it into a paste and set it aside to marinate for a bit. I then steam my face enough to open the pours, then apply my treatment. I leave it on for 15-20 minutes, then I rinse with a gentle homemade cleanser, then wipe with homemade baby wipes infused with frankincense. Your skin is going to feel baby soft and hydrated. The frankincense is also a soothing essential oil that compliments the collagen from the treatment. Turmeric works as a skin whitener and reverses the damage caused by toxins, rashes, and skin damage. This treatment is good to do anytime you feel your skin dehydrated, but for amazing results, use this treatment on your butterfly rashes and lesions. You'll be feeding your skin the food it's been longing for. One thing though, I'm not going to lie, this treatment smells terrible.

Food Sample Treatment #2

Honey and nutmeg. Honey is an antibacterial humectant

that benefits your skin by helping reduce the loss of moisture. Nutmeg is also antibacterial and great for breakouts, blemishes, rashes, and lesions.

Preparation

Mix one tbsp of honey to one tsp of nutmeg. Apply all over as a mask. Let dry. Then wash with warm water and a wash-cloth to help remove the treatment. Apply a small dollop of Jojoba oil as a moisturizer. This is a great winter and summer night hydration treatment as the winter and summer months are the most fragile seasons for Lupus skin.

Food Sample Treatment #3

A citrus and mint sugar scrub. Citrus fruits (whether you use lemon, limes, oranges, or grapefruits) are powerful healing skin treatments because they're loaded with vitamin C and citric acid. Vitamin C helps to reduce the delicate fine lines that develop from rashes and lesions on your face, while the citric acid gently burns away dark spots and blemishes. This burning sensation stimulates the body's natural self-healing defenses by encouraging collagen production, leaving your skin baby smooth. The sugar acts like an exfoliate, while the mint promotes a healing and cooling effect.

Preparation

Mix two tbsp of coconut oil with ½ cup of sugar. Add two tbsp of any citrus fruit zest of your choice. Add four drops peppermint essential oil, with two drops tea tree essential oil and scrub gently into skin. Always steam face before any treatment for better absorption of mixture.

Note

This treatment must NOT be done on skin currently in a rash or lesion flare up. The delicate nature of your skins condition will not be able to tolerate the harshness of the sugar scrubbing and may lead to additional abrasions on your skin that may turn into a bacterial skin infection.

Food Sample Treatment #4

An apple cider vinegar and green tea toner. This is a great mix for dark spot treatments as vinegar is an alpha hydroxy acid. After applying the vinegar, allow it to get absorbed into the skin and work its magic. Then spray a green tea and frankincense mist as an antioxidant skin toner.

Preparation

One cotton ball with apple cider vinegar, apply liberally on skin. In a small spray bottle add freshly brewed organic green tea. Let cool, then add two drops tea tree oil with two drops sweet orange oil.

Life-Style Healing Secret #3

A hydrotherapeutic facial blast. This is one of the most invigorating facial blasts to date. Hydrotherapy encourages blood flow and oxygen to the surface of the skin promoting healing and cell rejuvenation.

Preparation

In a pan boil water, place your face over the pan and cover your head with a towel. Gently blow the water to increase the amount of steam and heat if desired (if you have a facial steamer that would be ideal for safety purposes). Next, have already near you, a bowl that you can immerse your full face in comfortably, and fill it with ice and water. Steam your face for two minutes, then submerge your face in and out of the cold icy water for about one minute. Repeat this back and forth for about 20 minutes, no breaks. End on a hot cycle, let the skin dry naturally, then apply a small dollop of jojoba oil.

Note

If you're unable to tolerate the blast, then an alternative is to use freshly brewed tea bags and press them all over your face, then a cold spoon that is kept in your freezer and apply it on your skin. The timing for both the tea bags and the spoon is the same as above.

Life-Style Healing Secret #4

Red wine compress. This is fun for two reasons. Not only do you get to drink a glass of wine, but you also get to soak your face in it as well, talk about a win-win. The antioxidant and rejuvenating properties of red wine are an excellent source of polyphenols, resveratrol, and quercetin. So not only will you be looking healthier, but also, you'll be doing it in a heart healthy way while getting a nice buzz.

Preparation

In a bowl, add red wine. Take an absorbent paper towel and cut out lips and eyes. Now dip the mask in the wine and place it on your freshly steamed face. Sit back with some soothing music, a glass of wine and apply your mask. Continue to dip and apply for about thirty minutes. Then rinse, dry, and then apply your favorite moisturizer.

Note

For an even faster benefit, simmer the wine before dipping the towels, and then apply to your face. The steam from the wine feels AMAZING, and leaves your skin feeling so soft. I love applying a little jojoba oil after this treatment.

Healing Secret #5

Lymphatic drainage, facial exercises, and massages, are remedies sent from the gods. This has got to be the best and easiest natural facelift known to man. We never think of our skin as needing exercise and muscle toning. We were always taught to not be rough with our skin and to be gentle around the eyes.

This is far from the truth because the only way to promote collagen production and cell rejuvenation is to slightly injure the under layer of the skin, forcing the body to rejuvenate itself and heal the skin with more collagen and skin renewal.

At the end of the day, it is really important that we understand how critical it is to help the largest organ in our body system detox and expel toxins on a daily basis. Remember that Lupus begins to kill your organs and with the skin being an organ as well, we can't forget the importance of our skins need for nutrition and exercise. Through your skin you can reach all other organs. So, as we work from within flowing out, we should also work from the outside flowing in.

I have used these treatments on myself for years. I have also used them on my daughter, who also has Lupus, and every single one of my clients. That's how much I believe in these remedies.

CHAPTER 8
Strong Shiny Hair

"I am an amazing human being, living an incredibly blessed life. I am worthy of all things wonderful. I grow and learn each day. I let go of regrets from the past as they hold me there and prevent me from experiencing the now..."
~Carly Marie

Since my first Lupus episode, I have struggled with my hair. Every six months I would go through a hair growth spurt. It would look strong, healthy, shiny, then begin to grow like weeds. Then, suddenly, my hormones would go crazy and from one day to the next, clumps of hair would fall out and onto the shower floor. I basically got into the habit of practically shaving my head every five to six years. When they say that a woman's hair is her crown and glory, they weren't kidding. My Lupus hair has always made me feel like less than a woman because it was so delicate and fragile and unpredictable. But I have since come to peace with it as I have learned the secrets to growing out Lupus hair and reversing hair loss. I am excited for the many clients that have patiently allowed me to help them regrow their hair. The reviews on the treatments have been nothing but stellar and I'm so humbled when I get an email from a client telling me that their bald spots are beginning to fill in, or that they notice less hair falling out and their strands getting thicker.

However, even with that I'm not going to front, I have a long road ahead of me in completely getting over the mental and emotional damage my Lupus hair has caused me. As I mentioned before, my daughter also has Lupus, so I have made it my mission to apply treatments to her hair and make her love her frizz and curls. With my clients I work tirelessly to help them love their hair as well. I get so happy when I see my clients embrace their Lupus hair especially since you know the emotional damage it causes to their self-esteem. I'm so honored to be a part of their healing. So, without further ado, here are several of my favorite hair remedies for reducing Lupus hair-loss and regaining scalp strength and shine.

Hair-Loss Treatment (HLT)

HLT #1 ~Black Castor Oil

Black castor oil is an old ancient remedy for hair loss. It stimulates the hair follicles and promotes growth. It's excellent as a hot oil treatment and a leave-in conditioner. A little goes a long way so the best way to apply this remedy is with a small paint brush dipped in heated black castor oil. It's also fantastic in growing long beautiful lashes. This is a long-term solution that needs to be applied permanently to your beauty regime. In addition, castor oil is good as an antifungal for toenail fungus and helps grow beautiful strong nails. Castor oil is also used as a laxative and helps reduce burning in the gut. When ingested, it helps with skin and hair issues from within. My preference is Black Castor Oil, but if you find it too expensive, feel free to use regular castor oil. It's very important that you make sure that you're getting real castor oil; just stick to black castor oil from the health food store. Research your brands. Castor oil is also fantastic in bone broth smoothies. Just add one tablespoon and watch your body expel stuck on toxins living in your intestinal walls. You will start to see an increase in hair growth as you begin to eliminate stuck on mucoid plague and toxins from your intestines.

HLT #2 ~ Scalp Massager

An electric scalp massager is fantastic in bringing circulation to your scalp. Hydrotherapy is also fantastic for promoting hair growth as the extreme temperatures force oxygen into the scalp and work well with electric scalp massagers. It's always better to do these scalp circulation massages before you go to sleep, as your body will be free of stress, aiding in the relaxation of the scalp.

HLT #3 ~ Hair Masks

Another way of promoting the circulation of blood flow to the scalp is by using hair masks. One of my favorites is a black castor oil, honey, and crushed aspirin mask. Honey and black castor oil promote hair growth, as both also act as humectants that bring moisture to the hair and scalp, while the aspirin encourages the scalp to shed clogged pores and dandruff while promoting blood circulation to the scalp. This treatment can be very sticky so it's best to go light on the honey.

Another ingredient that can replace aspirin in this hair mask is the B3 vitamin niacin. Niacin will promote a niacin flush at the scalp, so if this is uncomfortable for you when taken as a supplement, keep in mind that this can also occur if used on the scalp as a hair mask as well. I don't mind it, in fact it's great for relieving headaches.

Another health promoting hair mask is the antibiotic promoting organic rice cream mask for hair and scalp. I have a video that shows exactly how to prepare this hair mask treatment on my Facebook page and other health promoting hair masks like this.

HLT #4 ~ Rice Water

Rice water is great for many uses. The water used to soak the rice is a natural antibiotic when fermented overnight. This water promotes hair growth when used as a hair rinse and hair tonic. It is also a great anti-wrinkle toner for the face and promotes healing from dandruff and psoriasis in the scalp.

In my videos, I will show you how to prepare hair and anti-aging tonics for your skin, scalp, and hair. Adding aloe gel, rose, or peppermint water is a great cooling tonic to add to the rice water for the summer months, to prevent scalp clogging which weakens hair follicles and increases hair thinning.

HLT #5 ~ Henna and oils

Henna is a wonderful hair-growth promoting herb. It protects and coats the hair and promotes thickness and density to hair follicles. Henna is great as a base when adding remedies that ignite its hair growing properties. There are many things you can add to your henna but my favorites are honey green tea instead of water as an antioxidant for the scalp and coffee to promote warm color. Essential oils are great additives that promote circulation and hair growth when combined with henna like tea tree, chamomile, peppermint, rosemary, ylang-ylang, lemon, eucalyptus, sweet orange, and frankincense just to name a few. Another additive that helps with the application of henna is aloe powder (juice or gel as well). Henna can be very stiff which can be difficult to apply on fine sensitive hair, but aloe smooths out the mask making it easier to apply to sensitive scalps and hair. It also nourishes and seals hair follicles. A great thing to do is to also add some aloe juice/gel and henna to your conditioner for that added body and color.

I'm thrilled that you got an opportunity to understand the benefits and remedies that are out there for Lupus hair. You don't have to feel helpless anymore because as long as there are natures organic healing foods still living on this planet, you will always have a treatment to help reverse Lupus hair.

CHAPTER 9
Weight Loss

*"Let Go... How would your life be different if you learned
to let go of things, that have already let go of you?"* ...
~Dr, Steve Maraboli

When it comes to weight loss and Lupus, that's a loaded topic, because most of the weight gain in Lupus sufferers is caused by toxic medications, lymphedema, inflammation of the organs, malfunctioning gall-bladder, and the body attacking itself and keeping the fat cells as hostage. Whether you look over-weight or anorexic, depending on your stage in this dis-ease, it has NOTHING to do with the calories in foods, but has A LOT to do with how your body reacts to the foods around you. It is very easy to become dehydrated when you have Lupus because everything you ingest should promote an anti-inflammatory response in your body. The increase of inflammation around your organs acts as a defense mechanism, which is where all the trouble begins, turning your metabolism on its head causing it to become sluggish and protective.

Below I'm going to list several of the usual suspects that are a good start for your new lifestyle remedies that, with their antioxidant properties, can aid in helping your digestion by promoting good gut health and anti-inflammatory responses without causing dehydration. It's critical that you NOT put yourself in the same box as other overweight people who do not have an autoimmune dis-ease. Our bodies function completely differently. Love yourself through your inflammatory weight-gain, just the same you would love yourself at your ideal weight. Your weight is between you and the universe, not between you and societies idea of what's attractive.

The "Me Now" Warrior Movement is about health and longevity. We are going to play by our own rules and create our own interpretation of beauty on a much broader scale that will love all shapes and sizes on this journey. We will celebrate keeping our weight, if we so desire, and we will encourage and support each other when we want to lose weight. All of this will be done through compassion, love, and empowerment. Like I mentioned before, your personal best will be a private relationship between you and the universe. I'll just be around as your human support.

First thing to consider before we begin is that we must become vigilant in picking our carbs. Now I'm not saying don't cheat because lord knows I do, but just remember to hold yourself accountable for both the good and the bad choices you make. Highly processed carbs, fats, and foods high in cholesterol, you know those highly sugary empty calorie delicious foods all around us that taste AMAZING, are the enemy of our immune system. Again, I'm not saying don't ever cheat, but what I am saying is that we need to know our bodies well enough to understand what will happen to us if we do tread in dangerous waters.

When we fall we must blame ourselves and not our condition. There is a long list of ways to eat the foods you love without them being processed, just like there are countless ways to satisfy your sweet tooth without it being unhealthy. Listen, I can't cook to save my life, but I have learned how to prepare essential healing foods from scratch with things that are readily available in my kitchen and didn't even know it. I want to teach you how to do the same. I also want to invite you to take a glimpse at a different food lifestyle that you can start immediately and self-pace to your own liking.

Achieving success or not achieving success in a healthy lifestyle change can be broken down into two very basic facts. You either seriously want to succeed, or you seriously "want to want" to succeed. One promotes healing and change, while the other feeds desire and blame. You can only hold on to desire and blame for so long. Not winning has to become exhausting for you before you decide it's time to embrace winning. The choice is up to you.

Anti-Inflammatory Remedies~#1

My number one favorite anti-inflammatory food that I never live without is broccoli. Broccoli is underrated and often taken for granted. Broccoli is a natural diuretic that promotes joint health and gut health, and aids in the elimination of parasites and toxins. It helps flush out fats and promotes weight loss. Because broccoli is high in vitamin K, it is said to help in the prevention of osteoarthritis and joint destruction. I remember in high school our ballet teacher insisting that we have a daily dose of broccoli. She knew how important it was to ensure that we girls did not have joint and bone damage due to osteoarthritis. I would recommend eating ALL parts of the broccoli as most of the nutrition is in the stem.

Anti-Inflammatory Remedies~#2

Organic dark leafy greens and fresh at home grown herbs like oregano, cilantro, parsley, basil, rosemary, thyme, and mint are a wonderful start to a clean new lifestyle. I love kale and baby spinach. These are known to be high in vitamin E and have high concentrated quantities of other important vitamins and powerful minerals. The best way to bring out these natural high potency nutrients, in all leafy greens, is to blanch them to make them easier for our bodies to digest. Aiding our gut to better digest food and better absorb their medicinal nutrients is key to transitioning smoothly into a new lifestyle.

Anti-Inflammatory Remedies~#3

An organic red juicy apple a day keeps the doctor away, and parasites, and inflammation, and helps flush out and regulate the bowels. Apples aid in gut health and kill cavity promoting bacteria in the mouth that can seep into our gut. They are also high in vitamins that help cleanse the skin from the inside out.

Anti-Inflammatory Remedies~#4

Choose purple foods, like blueberries and red cabbage. These colorful friends aid in brain and heart health. They are a great compliment to any food or drink and are a refreshing treat when included in a salad or if you're juicing.

Whether it be, purple, red, dark green, bright green, yellow, orange, or earthy colored medicinal foods, keeping colorful foods in their own color category helps bring out the richness of the vitamins, minerals, and properties their colors share in common.

Anti-Inflammatory Remedies~#5

Lastly, we have our orange power foods like sweet potatoes and carrots. These orange foods are high in beta-carotene and rich in vitamin C, E, and B. They're great for eye health along with skin, bones, and hair. Sweet potatoes are a great source of calcium and are a great substitute to white starchier potatoes.

There are literally hundreds of remedies that we can prepare with these and other super foods not mentioned here. Understanding the power of the nutrients in our foods and the combinations that can lead us to find our cure comes with patience, a fun team of friends, and a desire to step into our better selves. I look forward to healing forward with you soon.

PART FOUR:
Inspiring Recipes for Life

"Be gentle with your wounds. Be gentle with your heart.
You deserve to heal…"
~Dele Olunabi

CHAPTER 10

Medicinal Food Recipes 101 and Essential Oil Remedies

I n this final chapter I'd like to share a few delicious anti-inflammatory recipes that I've tried and had self-healing success with. These are recipes that my clients have rated as their top favorites for promoting healing in their self-care/self-love food list.

Note: Ingredients for foods and essential oils are listed, but please join our "MeNow" Warrior Movement Facebook group page for full recipes, preparations, and health properties. Join now cause your family and tribe await you with open arms.

Life-Style Inspiring Medicinal Food Recipe #1

Vegetable Kao Soi with Skinny Sweet Potato Fries

2 tbsp peanut oil

2 tbsp red curry paste

2 tsp curry powder

1 tsp turmeric

2 x 14 oz can coconut milk

1 cup bone broth or vegetable broth

1 whole star anise

1 cinnamon stick

1 tsp organic brown sugar

1 cup cauliflower florets

3 medium zucchinis

Juice of one lime

1 cup baby corn

Pink sea salt, to taste

Peppercorn to taste

To garnish, add one sweet potato julienned.

My client Jessica loved this recipe as she had just started becoming a vegetarian and felt lost. With this recipe she was able to use it as her base and just change the vegetables she wanted or leave out the curry for a cleaner and less spicy taste. Jessica started to embrace the feeling of self-empowerment she felt by becoming more in control of what she put in her body. This was her way of changing her story.

Life-Style Inspiring Medicinal Food Recipe #2

Black Bean and Vegetable chili

4 tbsp olive oil

2 onions chopped

2 red peppers chopped

3 roasted garlic cloves chopped

2 tbsp Chili powder

1 tbsp ground cumin

1 tbsp ground coriander

2 x 15 oz cans black beans

2 x 15 oz cans crushed tomatoes

¼ cup raw honey

¼ cup apple cider vinegar

1 ¾ cup frozen sweet corn

1-2 cups bone broth or vegetable stock

Alysa was always a fan of Mexican food but became afraid of eating out because of the heartburn and stomach pain she would experience after. This recipe allowed her to feel assured that the things going into her body were clean and on her list of remedies. After not getting any intestinal reactions to this Mexican favorite, Alysa was able to experiment with gluten free wraps that she baked and used as her dipping chips.

Life-Style Inspiring Medicinal Food Recipe #3

Eggplant and Okra Curry

2 large eggplants

1 tbsp vegetable oil

Chili paste

½ cup okra, cut into thirds

4 large tomatoes cut into wedges

1 ¾ cups canned coconut milk

Juice of a lime

1 large handful fresh cilantro leaves

Pink sea salt

Crushed peppercorn

Organic rice

Life-Style Inspiring Medicinal Food Recipe #4

Sweet potato, carrot, celery, and apple soup

1 lb shredded carrots blanched

2 unpeeled apples diced and blanched

2 tbs coconut oil, avocado, or MCT oil

1 shredded sweet potato

2 ½ cups bone broth (fresh or powdered)

1 clove roasted and smashed garlic.

½ tsp turmeric

½ tsp peppercorn grated

This is a gluten free post detox vitamin soup. One tbsp of healthy oils, like coconut oil, MCT oil, avocado oil, and within 10 days or sooner, will cut your joint pain as much as 50 percent. All are filled with antioxidants and rich nutrients that have inflammatory properties that calm an overactive painful nerves system.

These are just a few of the delicious recipes you will be experimenting with when you begin to build your own Lupus Recipe Checklist. All of these and other recipes in part five have been tested for negative Lupus reactions from clients and have been rated a high score on our "self-care/self-love healing scale". However, if you're currently having an issue with nightshades, it's best to avoid this recipe.

I only experience recipes that rate high on my self-care/self-love healing scale. What recipes will you find that will rate high on your self-healing scale?

Life-Style Inspiring Essential Oils

I wanted to end this chapter with a quick list of medicinal essential oils with their properties, treatments, and also give you an idea of how they can be used to promote healing for Lupus. It's a quick fun reference that you may turn to if you wish to include them into your beauty, nutritional cocktail, and/or medical food regimen. Enjoy!

Life-Style Essential Properties and Treatments

Essential oils and their powerful medicinal properties fall under several of healing categories. I like to stick with the ones that promote my AAOS regimen for healing. Learning these properties can give you a better feel for and understanding of how to use these oils on your Lupus self-healing journey.

Basil

Basil is a strong digestive aid and great for adding to your toothpaste as it aids in killing harmful bacteria in the mouth and gums. Basil is also good to use in a steam facial as it promotes healing for headaches and sinus infections.

Bergamot

Bergamot is another digestive aid that can also be applied to your toothpaste and also in your steam facials as it promotes healing of acne and is great in promoting skin health.

Black Pepper

Black pepper, another one for digestive aid, also helps in joint inflammation and pain as it carries strong anti-inflammatory properties.

Chamomile

Chamomile, another digestive aid (and an emotional and mental soothing aid), also falls under the property of an anti-inflammatory.

Sage

Sage is also a digestive aid that's fantastic for leaky gut syndrome. I make a mean Sage and Barley vitamin soup.

Sweet Orange

Sweet Orange is another one of my favorites as it soothes a nervous stomach. With its mild sedative properties, I like to apply to my toothpaste in the morning and let it absorb into my blood stream as a smooth calming treatment.

Peppermint

Peppermint is great for headaches, stomach upset, deodorant, appetite suppressant, mouthwash, and promotes scalp stimulation and hair growth.

Rosemary

Rosemary, another great hair elixir/tonic is also great for a fatty liver and inflammation of the organs. Very powerful.

Tea Tree

Tea Tree oil is fantastic as a skin tonic for all sorts of skin related issues. It is also fantastic at killing bacteria along with viruses associated with colds and flu. This is another treatment that can be added to a facial steam bath.

Eucalyptus

Eucalyptus is anti-viral and fantastic as an antiseptic for all sorts of cuts and wounds. I found that Eucalyptus also helps me with my Lupus fevers when I put them in my facial steam baths. It is also very calming.

Frankincense

Frankincense is probably on the top of my list as a Healer-Oil. Every morning and night, I apply a little dab on the roof of my mouth to eliminate any sinus pressure or headaches. Frankincense is a powerful anti-inflammatory that has been known to shrink tumors in the body.

Geranium

Geranium, like Tree Tea, is a very powerful antibacterial, antiseptic that promotes healing especially in skin lesions.

Ginger

Ginger is great for nausea and leaky gut. It promotes intestinal health and wellbeing. Take note that as an Ayurvedic remedy and tea, Ginger is rich in a rare plant compound called (zingibain) that releases and prevents the body from accumulating inflammation.

As a tea, Ginger is a diuretic with amazing healing properties; it helps release fluids relieving swelling, bloating, and water retention from lymphedema. Ginger will also help reduce pain and joint stiffness from rheumatoid and osteoarthritis.

Lemon

Lemon is a very powerful healer. It's fantastic for your immune system. As a tonic, if you don't have fresh organic lemons, just put several drops in your morning water routine and it becomes a great foundation for easing digestive issues in your gut and intestinal track. Add a little sweet orange to your water and you will be packing a powerful punch for your gut.

Myrrh

In biblical times Frankincense and Myrrh went hand in hand as THE most spiritual and powerful healing properties. Today it's no different. Myrrh promotes healing of the entire body system. It supports your immune system and is a fierce anti-inflammatory for Lupus inflamed organs.

Lavender

Lavender is great for soothing anxiety, depression and is great at promoting sound sleep. It has antibiotic and anti-inflammatory properties.

PART FIVE:
Inspiring Life Changing Journey

"When you feel like giving up remember why you started…"

~Healing Center

The "Me Now" Movement

A few years ago, I met a beautiful young girl named Hannah at the Tough Mudder challenge. I noticed that she walked the entire 12 miles and bypassed most of the 26 obstacles in the challenge. She was accompanied by her caretaker and grandmother who ran when Hannah ran, and walked when Hannah walked. We cordially waved at each other every so often during the race, I never thought much about it.

Now, what made me sign up for the race was that my doctor told me that my liver was in such bad shape that if I didn't go on the meds and see the other specialist he recommended, that I would be dead in a year because my body would be too septic to survive. So instead of listening to my doctors, I went sky diving and signed up for the Warrior Dash and the Tough Mudder Challenge. For those of you who have no idea what the Tough Mudder is, it is basically an excruciating 12-mile boot camp military challenge with 26 physically RIDICULOUS obstacles (like diving into a 16-feet-long, 6-feet-high dumpster full of water and ice cubes temped at 32-degrees, ***This was honestly my favorite obstacle and will be incorporating this into our "MeNow" Warrior Challenge next year), and of course the last obstacles, running through 20 feet of tightly spaced live electrical wires. So, you basically end the challenge electrocuted… Yum.

I went to this challenge as prepared as I possibly could be, wearing a t-shirt that read, "When my doctor said I had a year to live, I said f@#! IT! I'm doing the TOUGH MUDDER." Little did I know that Hannah was inspired by my t-shirt and signed up last minute at one of the late register booths. The reason I'm telling you this story is because Hannah, for a young girl, was in pretty bad shape. Hannah had stage IV Lupus and had been in and out of hospitals for the past three years when I met her. The reason she always came to sit by the sidelines is because five years prior to her diagnoses, she always did the Tough Mudder. She loved doing the Mudder and was in amazing shape before her diagnosis. She would always sit and watch the other challengers living the life she missed so much. When she saw me and read my t-shirt, she took it as the universe telling her to take one last turn at the Mudder and finish doing what she loved the most.

Coming close to the end of the finish line was Hannah and myself. We took so long that the afternoon challenge had already started and half of them had already reached the finish line. At the finish line I saw Hannah and her grandmother waiting for me at the exit. She introduced herself then told me her story and how much I had inspired her to not sit by the sidelines anymore. You see Hannah and I were kindred spirits because she and I both had Lupus. The difference being that she had been poorly diagnosed for the first three years and had been on so many meds that her fingers and toes were twisted from her arthritis. Her arms, legs, and face were scarred from her lesions and her prognosis was not good. We were both given a death sentence except she had reached the point of no return.

The three of us spoke for a good hour and I made Hannah a promise. I told her that one day I would create a challenge similar to the Tough Mudder for Lupus patients surviving at all stages of the dis-ease. A "MeNow" Warrior Challenge representing our fight, our journey, and our healing. Well I am blessed to say that this book is the beginning of that dream, that promise that I made four years ago. I never told anyone this story because I never knew if it could ever happen, so I just put it on my bucket list and went on with my life.

Now you have heard my story and got a glimpse of what I use to heal myself and my clients from this so called, "incurable" condition and auto-immune dis-ease we call Lupus. I refuse to accept the "incurable" diagnosis part and I hope you do as well.

We are only incurable when we don't get the right cure, not because we're doomed because of our condition. I know that there are a host of scientifically backed and proven organic natural foods and remedies that can reverse the symptoms of organ failure, joint and muscle deterioration, and heart disease and I'm inviting you to ride along the remission train with me.

Here's to healing forward together…. Cheers!

Acknowledgments

I n my many moments of solitude, ever since I can remember, the universe has been my best friend, my mentor, and guide. I have always had many extraordinary experiences, however, there were times when my distractions and outside noises failed me, and I missed these opportunities.

In these moments, I've always heard the universe say, in its loving soothing voice, "We can sit in this darkness for a little while longer, but wouldn't you rather see what we can create on the other side of this sadness?" I would hear, "Visualize where you would like to go next. Wouldn't you like to be there now?" Every time I felt myself falling into that dark hole of despair, I would trust these moments and say, "Yes, I want to see what's on the other side," and no matter how much my body couldn't move, and as foggy as my eyes would see, and as groggy as my mind would be, I knew I would be crossing over into another

"Me Now" Warrior moment that would push me ten steps further ahead on my journey.

I want to thank the universe for all the rewarding life-changing and character-building experiences that continue to guide me as I grow into a better version of myself. I especially want to thank Divine Mind for the many amazing, and not so amazing, people I have met on my journey who have come to me as either life lessons or clues directing me towards my life's hidden treasure.

To the Morgan James Publishing team: Special thanks to David Hancock, CEO & Founder for believing in me and my message. To my Author Relations Manager, Gayle West, thanks for making the process seamless and easy. Many more thanks to everyone else, but especially Jim Howard, Bethany Marshall, and Nickcole Watkins.

Thank you Angela Lauria, my sista-from-anotha-motha, for being the answer and truly the dream come true for all our Ideal Readers. To the whole Incubating Team, for keeping everything flowing smoothly and on track. To my Quill family, I love how even though we are all at different stages of success in our journeys, we're all in the divine learning process together. Thank you, Cheyenne, for being such a beacon of light and calm for all us drama queens. Thank you to an amazing marketing team and especially my incredibly amazing marketing manager and editor

Cynthia Kane, she really gets me and helped me nail this for my Ideal Reader.

Blessings

About the Author

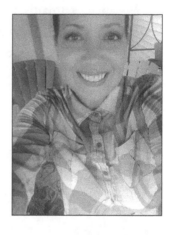

WiseBetty specializes in helping Lupus and autoimmune clients. She started her "Me Now" Warrior Movement as a promise to a friend to help other autoimmune and Lupus patients walk into their better selves through community, empowerment, knowledge, determination, joy, patience and love. She has spent most of her life experimenting with organic ancient remedies, natural medicinal foods and supplemental properties to help eliminate her Lupus symptoms while on a self-healing mission. She is very passionate about helping her clients create a healthier more satisfying life both mentally and physically.

WiseBetty is excited to be able to bring her knowledge, and life's experiences and share it with the world through her books, seminars, speaking engagements, her "MeNow" Self-Healing Retreats and her "MeNow" Warrior Challenges, what she likes to call her "Movements of Self-Empowerment and Healing."

WiseBetty currently resides in upstate New York and the Poconos with her daughter and three kids with paws. She loves spending time experimenting with new remedies, dedicating herself to her studies, creating art and dance, and sipping fine wine with friends.

Thank You!

Thank you so much for reading my book, and thank you for being an advocate for yourself and your health. The fact that you've gotten this far in the book shows me that you're ready for change. You're ready to live a pain free life again. You're choosing to experience and embrace self-healing and a joy for life, and for that, I respect you. Accepting my invitation to join the "Me Now" movement is the beginning of a life changing and worthwhile journey into your better and healthier self and I'm honored that you're putting your trust in me. And because of your commitment, I have now become your biggest fan, your #1 cheerleader.

To support you in starting your healing on the right foot, I created the **"Me Now" Self-Healing Call-to-Action Checklist** just for you. It's a **FREE** simple diagnostic assessment to help you get crystal-clear on how you plan on succeeding on your self-healing journey. We'll evaluate which physical obstacles we'll need to address and what self-limiting narrative we'll need to help you overcome.

You can get your **FREE** copy of the **"Me Now" Self-Healing Call-to-Action Checklist** by sending your request to the-menowmovement@groups.facebook.com

One more thing, if you enjoyed this book, a great way to express your gratitude is to write a review. When you get the book (and the secret surprise you'll receive once you've joined and taken the **"Me Now" Self-Healing Call-to-Action Checklist**), be sure to drop a review on Amazon and/or post a picture of yourself holding the book on Facebook or Instagram!

Facebook https://www.facebook.com/groups/themenowmovement/

Instagram https://www.instagram.com/mastershay1/

This is going to be an absolutely amazing self-healing adventure. So, bust out your journals and your journey shoes, click to join the movement, and let's get this party started.

Printed in the USA
CPSIA information can be obtained
at www.ICGtesting.com
JSHW082358140824
68134JS00020B/2138